CANCER AND MODERN SCIENCE™

LUNG CANCER

Current and Emerging Trends in Detection and Treatment

JULIE WALKER

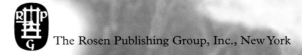

The Rosen Publishing Group, Inc., New York

Published in 2006 by The Rosen Publishing Group, Inc.
29 East 21st Street, New York, NY 10010

Copyright © 2006 by The Rosen Publishing Group, Inc.

First Edition

Library of Congress Cataloging-in-Publication Data

Walker, Julie.
Lung cancer: current and emerging trends in detection and treatment/
by Julie Walker.—1st ed.
    p. cm.—(Cancer and modern science)
ISBN 1-4042-0388-5 (library binding)
1. Lungs—Cancer—Juvenile literature.
I. Title. II. Series.
RC280.L8W34 2006
616.99'424—dc22

                                                                2004025554

Manufactured in Malaysia

On the cover: Photograph of cancerous lung tissue cells, magnified 900 times.

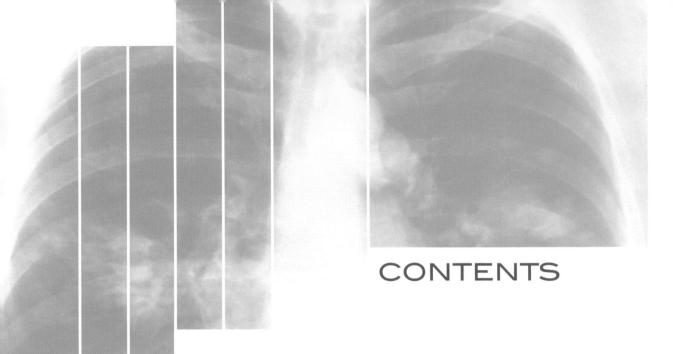

CONTENTS

INTRODUCTION

Believe it or not, the most frequently diagnosed form of cancer in the United States is also the most preventable. According to the World Health Organization, lung cancer is currently the leading cancer killer among men and women in the United States and worldwide. The American Cancer Society predicts that by the end of 2005, about 172,570 new cases of lung cancer will be diagnosed in the United States and more than 160,000 people will die from the disease.

The leading risk factor for developing lung cancer is cigarette smoking. Approximately 87 percent of lung cancer deaths occur as a result of exposure to cancer-causing chemicals, called carcinogens, found in tobacco. Because this risk factor far outweighs any other, scientists are currently working on different techniques to help people quit smoking and also to prevent people from starting in the first place. Scientists are also conducting investigations into the many other risk factors for lung cancer, including exposure to radon gas and a person's heredity and diet. Still other researchers are testing new methods for diagnosing lung cancer earlier so that victims can live longer, healthier lives.

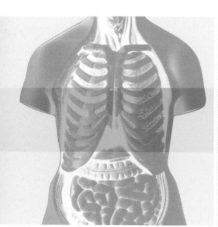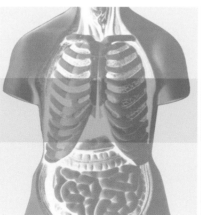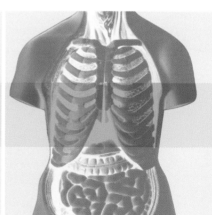

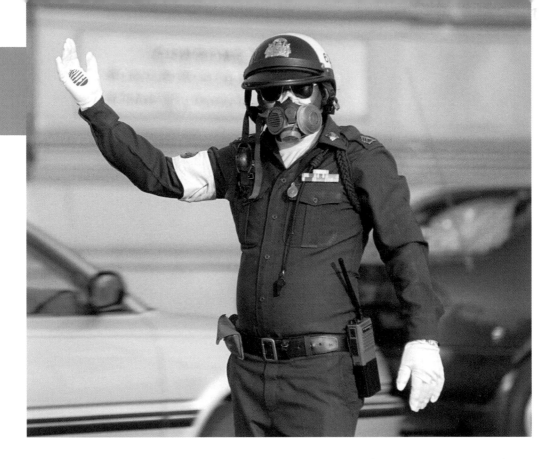

Although cigarette smoking is the number one cause of lung cancer, nonsmokers are at risk as well. People exposed to secondhand smoke, asbestos, or radon are in danger of developing lung cancer. Another cause of the disease is exhaust from diesel fuel used in many buses and trucks. Here, a traffic policeman wears a mask to avoid pollutants that could cause him to develop lung problems.

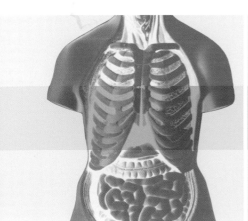
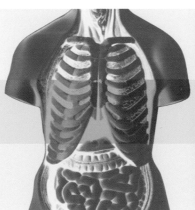
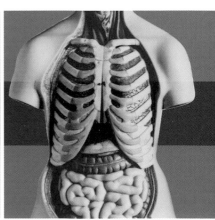

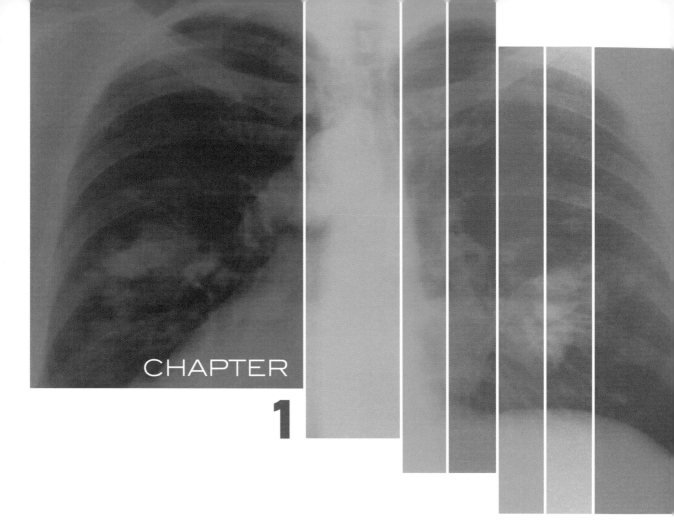

WHAT IS LUNG CANCER?

The human body is made up of trillions of cells. Most of these cells regularly go through a process of dividing, called mitosis, in order to replace worn-out or damaged cells. Every time a healthy cell divides, two new cells are created, each identical to the original cell. This process of cell reproduction is absolutely essential for the proper operation of all the tissues, organs, and systems at work in our bodies.

Occasionally, however, something causes mitosis to go haywire. Why might healthy cells suddenly behave in such a strange way?

Exposure to a carcinogen, a cancer-causing substance, may damage the genetic material found inside a cell. As soon as a normal cell "recognizes" that this material, called DNA (deoxyribonucleic acid), is damaged, it will either fix the problem or die. In a cancer cell, however, the abnormal DNA cannot be repaired and will continue to reappear in every new cancer cell. These cancer cells begin to divide at an abnormally rapid rate, and soon, a large mass of cells forms. This cluster of cells is referred to as a tumor.

Tumors are classified as either benign or malignant. A benign tumor is not life threatening and will not spread to other parts of the body. The cells that make up a malignant tumor are classified as cancer cells. Cancer cells grow and reproduce at a rapid rate and are able to live longer than normal cells. They are also capable of breaking off from their original site and traveling to other parts of the body, which is referred to as metastasis. Often, cancer cells take a speedy, direct route to other organs by entering the bloodstream.

CANCER IN THE LUNGS

According to the American Lung Association, lung cancer accounts for 14 percent of all types of cancers and 28 percent of all cancer-related deaths. In many cases, lung cancer begins in the cells lining the bronchi, but it may also begin in the trachea, bronchioles, or alveoli. The original tumor that forms from cancer cells is referred to as the primary tumor.

Although other types of lung cancer do exist, most lung cancer cases can be divided into two major groups based on the type of cells found in the primary tumor: small cell lung cancer (SCLC) and non-small cell lung cancer (NSCLC). Once a tumor is detected, cells in the primary tumor must be carefully identified under a microscope in order to correctly distinguish between these two types of lung cancer. This is very important because SCLC and NSCLC grow and spread in different ways, and they respond differently to cancer treatments. Physicians must clearly diagnose the type of cancer before determining a plan of treatment.

LUNG ANATOMY AND FUNCTION

The lungs are two spongy organs that take up most of the space in your chest. The right lung consists of three lobes, or sections, and the left lung consists of two lobes. The left lung is smaller than the right lung due to the location of the heart. A protective, moist lining called the pleura surrounds the lungs. The pleura allows the lungs to expand and contract easily as you breathe.

The lungs are the central organs of the respiratory system. The first basic function of the respiratory system is breathing. The lungs bring air in and out of the body every time you inhale and exhale. Air travels down the trachea, or windpipe, into tubes called the bronchi. The bronchi split,

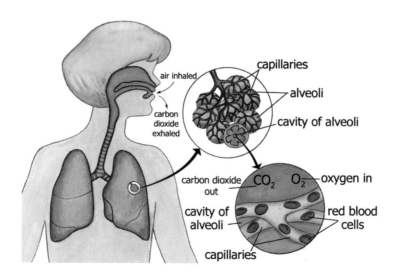

Deep within the lungs, one of the most vital chemical reactions takes place. Respiration involves the transfer of oxygen and carbon dioxide across the capillaries winding through the alveoli. This exchange of gases is essential for survival.

allowing air to enter the right and left lungs and then divide further into smaller tubes called the bronchioles. At the very end of each bronchiole are tiny air sacs called alveoli.

It is in the alveoli that the next major function of the respiratory system takes place. About one billion tiny blood vessels called capillaries wind their way through the alveoli. This is where the chemical reaction of respiration takes place. Oxygen from the inhaled air is absorbed into the bloodstream. All the cells in the body depend on oxygen to properly function. When oxygen combines with glucose, a simple sugar produced by cells, energy is released. Cells require this energy to be able to do their various jobs within the body. At the same time, carbon dioxide is released from the cells and travels back through the bloodstream to the lungs. Exhaling carbon dioxide is also essential for healthy cells since too much can be deadly. When the health of the lungs is compromised, the entire body is at risk.

SMALL CELL LUNG CANCER

SCLC accounts for approximately 20 to 25 percent of all lung cancers. Although the cells found in this type of lung cancer are small, they are able to grow and multiply very quickly. This unique characteristic is the reason scientists group SCLC separately from NSCLC. Due to such rapid cell growth, large tumors form quickly and are usually located in the bronchi or near the center of the lungs. In addition to growing aggressively in the lungs, SCLC spreads to other parts of the body early. Often, the cancer cells have spread even before the patient notices any symptoms of the disease.

Tobacco smoking causes almost all cases of SCLC. In fact, according to the Alliance for Lung Cancer Advocacy, Support, and Education

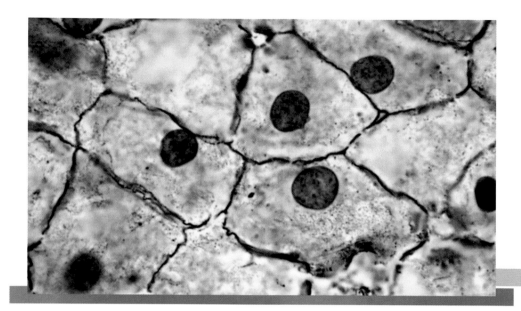

The second-most common type of lung cancer, squamous cell carcinoma, is a type of non-small cell lung cancer. The image above shows a magnification of squamous cells, identified by their resemblance to fish scales. On an X-ray, one method of detection, a squamous cell carcinoma appears as a shaded area. Squamous cell carcinomas usually develop in the central portions of the lungs.

(ALCASE), only about 1 percent of small cell lung cancer occurs in people who have never smoked. Because SCLC is characterized by rapid cell growth and metastasis, patients usually have a poor prognosis. The American Lung Association reports the average survival rate of a patient diagnosed with SCLC to be only thirty-five weeks.

NON–SMALL CELL LUNG CANCER

NSCLC accounts for approximately 75 to 80 percent of all lung cancers. This type of lung cancer has been divided into three categories: squamous cell carcinoma, adenocarcinoma, and large cell carcinoma. These three types of lung cancer are grouped together because of similarities in their cell growth and the way they are treated.

Squamous cell carcinoma accounts for about 25 to 30 percent of all lung cancers. This type of cancer is the most common form found in men, especially those who smoke. Squamous cells are large and flat. They are usually found in tumors near the center of the lung area, near the bronchi. Unlike their small cell counterparts, squamous cells grow slowly. In fact, these cells may stay in the lung region for long periods of time before spreading to other organs. This quality gives squamous cell carcinoma patients a more favorable prognosis than those with SCLC. In fact, more than half will survive at least five years after their diagnosis of squamous cell carcinoma.

Adenocarcinoma accounts for approximately 35 to 40 percent of all lung cancers. This is the most common type of lung cancer in women, in people who have never smoked, and in people younger than age fifty. While the number of squamous cell carcinoma cases has decreased over the past thirty years, the frequency of adenocarcinoma has increased. Until recently, adenocarcinoma was less common than squamous cell carcinoma in the United States. Currently, scientists are researching possible reasons for this increase. Ideas include changes in diet, smoking habits (70 percent of those diagnosed with adenocarcinoma are smokers), and environmental factors.

Adenocarcinoma cells are shaped like cubes or columns. Tumors are most often detected in the outer edges of the lung or under the lining of the bronchi. Masses of the adenocarcinoma cells look and behave like glands. Like a gland, most adenocarcinoma tumors are able to produce and release a thick liquid called mucin. Compared to the other types of lung cancer, adenocarcinoma has an average rate of cell growth and spreading. Less than 10 percent of patients with adenocarcinoma are expected to live five years after their diagnosis.

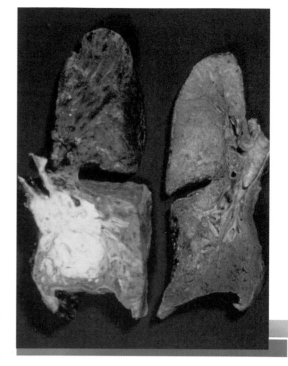

This photograph proves that there is a visible difference between a fairly healthy lung (right) and a lung diseased by cancer (left). Note the white spot on the lower lobe of the cancerous lung, indicating a tumor. The upper lobe has been blackened by a longtime and heavy cigarette habit. The lung on the right, while healthy, does show signs of some damage, perhaps from light cigarette use or minimal exposure to environmental carcinogens.

The final type of NSCLC is the large cell undifferentiated carcinoma, which accounts for only 10 to 15 percent of all lung cancers. As the name implies, these are the largest cells of all the categories of NSCLC. The term "undifferentiated" means that the cells are quite immature. Their structure and functions are simpler than the squamous cells or adenocarcinoma cells.

While large cell undifferentiated carcinoma is not limited to one location, tumors are commonly found in the smaller bronchi. This type of lung cancer also grows more rapidly and spreads earlier than the other types of NSCLC. As a result, less than 10 percent of patients diagnosed with large cell undifferentiated carcinoma are expected to live longer than five years.

BEYOND THE LUNGS

If cancer cells spread, the tumors they create in other parts of the body are called secondary, or metastastic, tumors. The natural pathways

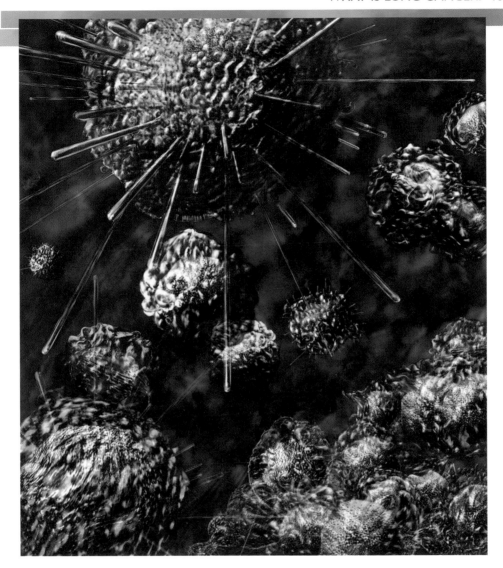

A cancerous tumor can spread, or metastasize, from the lungs and invade other organs in the body. This illustration depicts a collection of replicated cells that have formed a tumor at the lower right corner. Some cells have broken off from the tumor and floated away. The large cell at the upper left radiates projections that help it move through blood and lymph vessels and attach to surfaces. One of the dangers of lung cancer is that, because there are very few symptoms for a patient to notice, tumors that originate in the lungs often go undetected until they have metastasized to other parts of the body.

for cells to travel from one organ to another are the blood or lymph vessels. Secondary tumors that originated in the lungs often will develop in the brain, bone, liver, and bone marrow. Metastastic lung cancer is the term that refers to any lung cancer that has spread beyond the lungs.

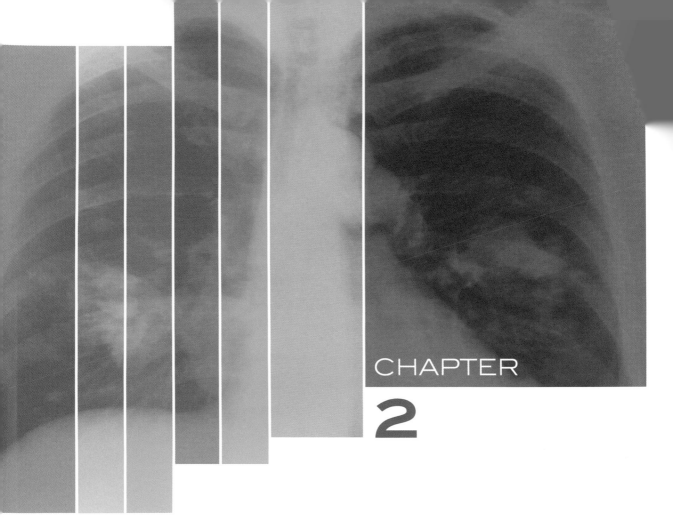

RISK FACTORS: WHAT CAUSES LUNG CANCER?

A risk factor is anything that increases a person's chance of developing a disease such as lung cancer. Each of the risk factors for lung cancer can produce changes in the DNA of the lung cells. These changes, or mutations, can cause the cells to become cancerous. Although the leading cause of lung cancer is cigarette smoke, there are many other factors that may put a person at risk for developing lung cancer. Proof of this lies in the numbers: only one out of every ten people who smoke cigarettes develops lung cancer, and one out of every six people with lung cancer has never smoked!

HISTORY OF LUNG CANCER

Lung cancer is a relatively new disease. Cigarette manufacturing began as early as the 1880s, but it was not until the United States entered World War I (1914–1918) that smoking this sort of tobacco product became popular in American culture. Soldiers were offered free cigarettes (which, unlike pipes, cigars, and chewing tobacco, contained hundreds of chemicals) from the tobacco companies, and the habit continued when they returned home. At that time, of course, no one understood the long-term health effects of the carcinogens found in cigarette smoke.

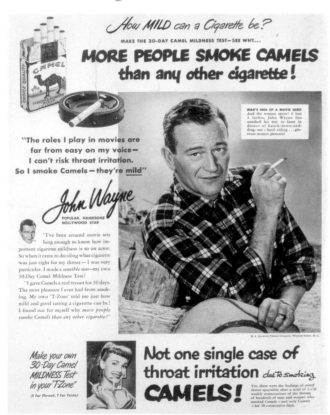

It's hard to believe, but there was a time when cigarettes were widely advertised in magazines and on television. This 1950 ad shows Western movie legend John Wayne endorsing Camel cigarettes. Celebrities regularly promoted cigarettes for decades, lending to the public's perception that smoking was glamorous. By the 1990s, the only advertisements showing cigarettes were public service announcements warning that cigarette smoking was potentially deadly.

Because no one expected smoking to produce such deadly results and because symptoms of lung cancer may take years to appear, doctors did not notice a dramatic increase in the number of lung cancer cases until the 1930s. Researchers responded to the epidemic, and by the 1950s, a link between the increase in cigarette smoking and the increased number of lung cancer patients was apparent.

At the time when cigarette smoking became prevalent in the United States, it was mostly men who smoked. Therefore, when lung cancer diagnosis began to increase, it was men who had the disease. Over time, as more and more women began to smoke, the cases of lung cancer in women increased as a result. In the thirty years from 1962 to 1992, the number of women diagnosed with lung cancer increased by 550 percent. In 1987, lung cancer actually surpassed breast cancer as the leading killer of women. Today, lung cancer is responsible for more deaths every year in the United States than breast, colon, and prostate cancer combined.

SMOKING TOBACCO PRODUCTS

According to the American Lung Association, cigarette smoking accounts for approximately 87 percent of deaths caused by lung cancer. In other words, seven out of eight people who die from lung cancer are either current or former smokers. Many of the chemicals found in cigarettes have been studied by scientists and classified as carcinogens. One of the chemicals found in tobacco is nicotine, an addictive drug. Because people who smoke become addicted to nicotine, it is very difficult for them to stop smoking.

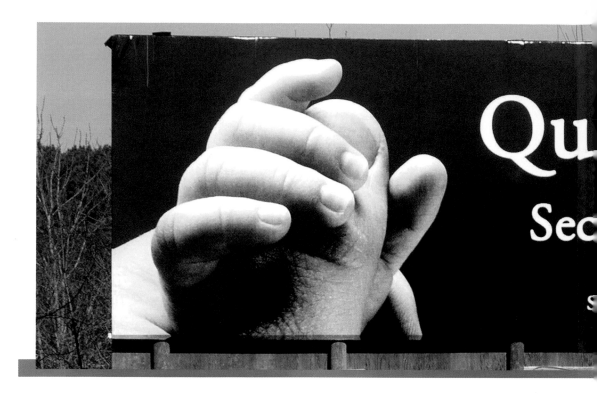

To claim that smoking tobacco products is a risk factor for lung cancer is a bit too simple, because many other variables exist. For example, research has shown that there is a strong connection between the age at which a person begins to smoke and the likelihood that he or she will develop lung cancer. Smoking at a younger age raises the risk of lung cancer. The total number of years a person smokes is also a risk factor. The dangerous effects of carcinogens found in tobacco smoke have been proven to accumulate, or add up, over time. In addition, the number of cigarettes smoked per day is a factor. When some of these variables are considered together, the term "total lifetime exposure" may be used. Take two smokers: One smokes ten cigarettes a day for ten years, while the other smokes twenty cigarettes a day for five years. Both individuals have an equal

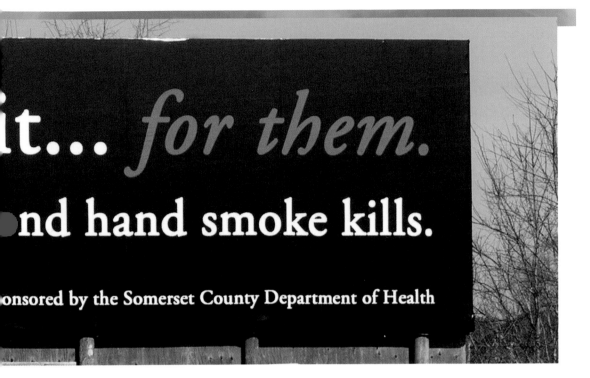

This billboard points out the fact that a person's decision to smoke affects people other than the smoker. The most frequent victims of secondhand smoke are children, whose lungs are still developing and can be permanently disabled by the poisons from cigarette smoke. Secondhand smoke in the home can even cause pets to develop lung cancer.

total lifetime exposure and, therefore, may be at the same risk for developing lung cancer. There are, however, many other risk factors to consider.

EXPOSURE TO SECONDHAND SMOKE

Secondhand smoke is the vapor and fumes released from a lit tobacco product or exhaled from a smoker. A person exposed to secondhand smoke is a nonsmoker who is in the company of one or more smokers.

He or she inhales the smoke from a nearby cigarette and becomes indirectly exposed to the carcinogens found in tobacco smoke.

In 1986, the surgeon general officially reported research findings linking secondhand smoke to lung cancer. In 1992, the Environmental Protection Agency reported that secondhand smoke leads to about 3,000 cases of lung cancer each year in the United States. Secondhand smoke may also be referred to as environmental smoke, passive smoke, or sidestream smoke (the opposite of mainstream smoke, which is inhaled directly into the lungs from a cigarette).

EXPOSURE TO RADON

Radon is a gas that is sometimes found in soil, rocks, groundwater, and building materials. It is a radioactive element and a proven carcinogen. Breathing air that contains high levels of radon increases a person's risk for developing lung cancer. The American Lung Association reports that radon is the second leading cause of lung cancer in the United States and accounts for about 10,000 deaths each year. Twelve percent of all lung cancer deaths can be linked to radon.

The problem for people arises when radon is present indoors. If radon is produced underneath a building, the gas may creep inside through gaps or cracks in the basement or through pipes, drains, or similar openings. Also, if radon is present in the groundwater where a well exists, the gas can be released into the air when people shower or use water indoors for other reasons. Research shows that radon entering a home through the soil presents a much greater risk than radon entering through water. Although rare, it is possible for a person to develop stomach cancer from ingesting, or swallowing, water with high levels of radon.

Because radon gas is completely invisible and odorless, people living or working in a building with high radon levels may be completely unaware that they are in danger. The Environmental Protection Agency

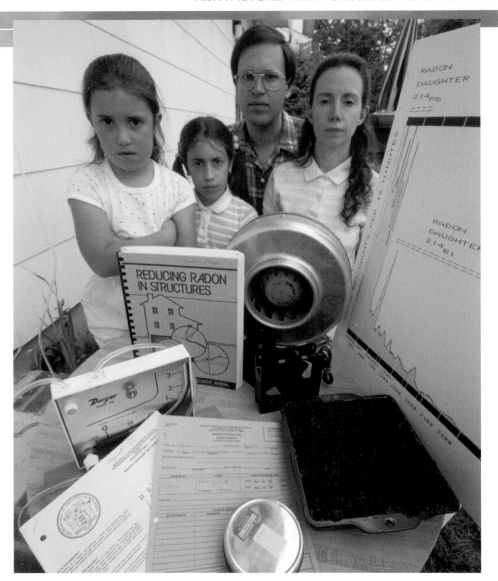

Radon is known as the "silent killer" because it cannot be seen or smelled. Most people don't know if it is present in their home or workplace until they test for radon levels. The good news is that home owners and landlords are aware of the dangers of radon, and are installing detectors in buildings. Also, new structures are being built with radon levels in mind. The family in this photograph is planning on constructing their new home with attention to reducing radon levels within the structure.

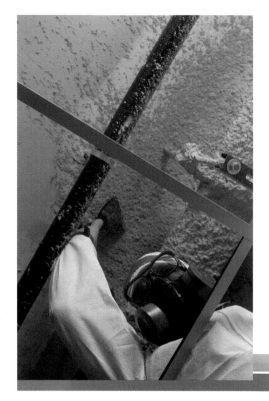

A natural mineral widely used for building insulation and as a fire retardant, asbestos was discovered in the mid-20th century to be a carcinogen. Most people didn't develop asbestos-related lung cancer until about twenty years after being exposed to the material, so it continued to damage lungs for decades. Now, asbestos usually is found only in older buildings. If exposed, it needs to be repaired or removed, as shown in this photograph.

estimates that approximately one out of every fifteen homes has radon levels at or above acceptable levels.

EXPOSURE TO OTHER CARCINOGENS

Quite a few substances in addition to tobacco and radon have been studied and determined to be carcinogens for lung cancer. Two stand out as more common: asbestos and diesel exhaust.

At one time, asbestos was frequently used in building materials such as insulation. It quickly became evident that people exposed to asbestos either in their workplace or in their home were at a greater risk for lung cancer. Asbestos causes a particular kind of cancer called mesothelioma, which often begins in the pleura, the outer covering of the lung. Asbestos workers are, in fact, seven times more likely to die from lung cancer than someone not exposed. Due to the close link between exposure to asbestos and lung cancer, the U.S. government

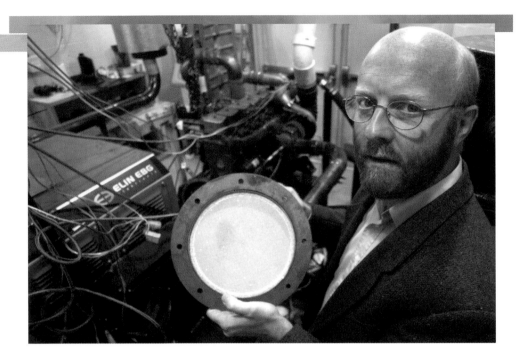

Research is being conducted to eliminate pollution from diesel engines and gasoline-powered cars, which can lead to lung cancer. Here, an employee of Corning, Inc., displays a diesel particulate filter the company is testing. Such filters could cut down on tens of thousands of premature deaths each year.

has nearly banned its use in the workplace and in products for the home.

Although the risk may not be as great as exposure to asbestos, long-term exposure to the chemicals in the exhaust of diesel engines most likely causes lung cancer. In the year 2007, laws requiring trucks and buses to upgrade diesel exhaust systems will begin to go into effect.

Additionally, the risk of lung cancer is multiplied if a person has been exposed to more than one carcinogen. For example, a smoker who is exposed to asbestos is more likely to develop lung cancer than a smoker who is not exposed to asbestos.

POTENTIAL LUNG CANCER GENE DISCOVERED

Researchers have recently discovered a possible link between lung cancer and heredity. The Genetic Epidemiology of Lung Cancer Consortium (GELCC) analyzed the genetic makeup of fifty-two families, each of which had at least three members affected by the disease. Scientists found evidence that a gene or genes making a person more susceptible to lung cancer is located on chromosome 6. Thousands of genes are located on each of a human body cell's forty-six chromosomes. The next step for researchers is to conduct experiments that will pinpoint the exact location of the gene or genes responsible for susceptibility to lung cancer. The GELCC scientists also studied the effect of smoking on people with or without the lung cancer gene. Their findings indicate that smoking even a little can lead to cancer in people with the lung cancer gene. The results of the study were published in the September 2004 issue of the *American Journal of Human Genetics*.

HEREDITY

Heredity is the passing on of traits from parents to offspring, from one generation to the next. Whether lung cancer is hereditary is a topic of current research. Genes are responsible for controlling how cells handle exposure to carcinogens, for example. They also may determine how well the cells in the immune system detect and destroy cancer cells. If a mutation, or change, occurs in one of these genes, the cells will not receive the proper instructions. One specific

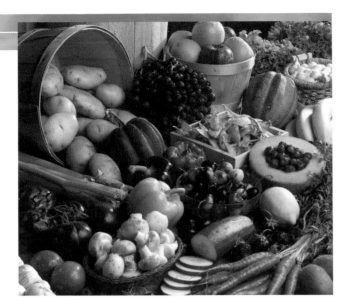

Though researchers have not pinpointed exactly which foods can help prevent lung cancer, they do know that a diet rich in fruits and vegetables that contain antioxidants and certain vitamins can lower a person's risk of developing lung cancer.

mutation has been discovered in a gene located on chromosome 19 (every human body cell contains forty-six chromosomes, each containing thousands of genes). This particular gene contains the code for making a protein that scientists believe to be a tumor suppressor. This means that the protein stops a tumor from either forming in the first place or from multiplying and growing larger. If the cells do not receive the message to make this protein, or if it is made incorrectly, the tumors will not be suppressed. The result in this case is lung adenocarcinoma.

DIET

The role that diet plays as a risk factor for developing lung cancer is currently being researched. Some reports suggest that a diet low in certain fruits and vegetables may place a person at a greater risk. It may be possible that vitamins A and E contain a substance capable of protecting the body from lung cancer. That means that eating fruit and green and yellow vegetables may decrease the risk of lung cancer. Much more research is necessary to test this hypothesis.

OTHER DISEASES

The final risk factor for lung cancer affects people who have already had other diseases such as tuberculosis or certain forms of pneumonia. Both of these diseases may cause the lungs to become inflamed, or swollen. This inflammation may then result in the formation of scars on the lungs. Scientists believe that scarring of the lung tissue may increase a person's chances of developing lung cancer.

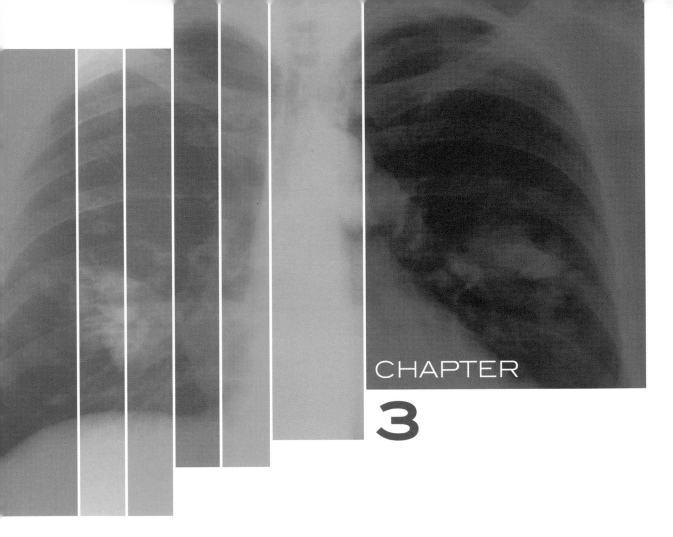

SYMPTOMS AND DIAGNOSIS OF LUNG CANCER

One of the frightening facts about lung cancer is that it is rarely caught in its early stages. Only 15 percent of all lung cancer cases are detected before the cancer has spread to other parts of the body. Sometimes the cancer is found incidentally, perhaps from a chest X-ray that was taken for another reason. Other times, however, a patient goes to his or her doctor with early symptoms, which vary a great deal. This variation is due to the location and size of the tumor and the involvement of different lymph nodes in different locations.

The most common symptom of people with lung cancer in the early stages, before the cancer spreads, is a persistent cough. Over half of the people diagnosed with lung cancer have complained of a cough. In the case of a nonsmoker, the cough is new. A current smoker, on the other hand, may notice a change in an existing cough.

The following symptoms are less common, but may occur in a person diagnosed in the early stages of lung cancer.

— Chest pain
— Shortness of breath
— Hoarseness
— Coughing up blood (hemoptysis)
— Difficult and/or painful breathing
— Unintentional weight loss
— Fatigue (exhaustion)
— Bloody or brown sputum (spit or phlegm)
— Fever
— Repeated lung infections such as bronchitis or pneumonia

A tumor may reach the advanced stages of lung cancer before metastasizing to other organs. In those cases, the tumor is large enough to begin affecting structures on or near the lungs. The specific location of the tumor directly affects the symptoms the patient experiences. A new or different hoarseness in a person's voice may mean that the tumor is pressing on the nerves near his or her vocal cords. Difficulty swallowing may indicate a tumor pressing on the esophagus (the tube that brings food from the mouth to the stomach). Shoulder pain or numbness in an arm or hand may result from a tumor in the upper part of the lungs. A person's face may swell due to a tumor pressing on a

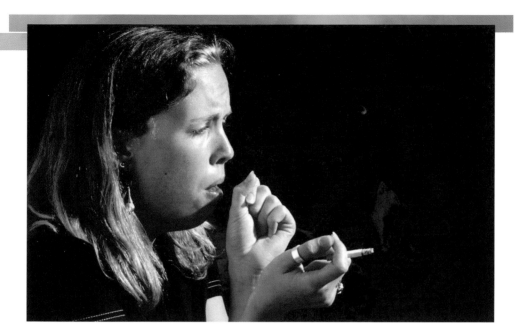

Cigarette smoking has many side effects, including a persistent cough and compromised lung function. People who begin a smoking habit in their teens stand a greater chance of developing lung cancer. Since nicotine is addictive, it is better not to start at all.

vein leading to the heart. Because the tumor could be anywhere on any of the lobes of the lungs, the variety of symptoms seems endless.

Unfortunately, most people are diagnosed long after the cancer has metastasized to distant organs of the body. Secondary tumors are referred to as metastases. Although cancer that originates in the lungs can spread to any organ, the most common sites are the brain, liver, and bones. Brain metastases, for example, refer to secondary tumors located in the brain that originated in the lungs. A person with brain metastases may experience severe headaches, vomiting, and seizures. Depending on the specific location of the tumor, a person's motor control (ability to move), vision, speaking, balance, and ability to focus may be affected. Bone metastases are usually associated with pain, especially when the pain is not connected to an injury of any sort. Liver metastases also result in severe pain. The liver is contained in a cavity with little room to spare, so as a tumor on it grows, the pressure on the liver increases. The fact that so few cases of lung cancer are found before metastases occur is the reason that this disease is so devastating.

METHODS OF DETECTION

When a patient brings any of the above symptoms to the attention of a physician, the doctor's job is to determine whether cancer is present. There are certain steps in the diagnosis of lung cancer that a doctor will follow, beginning with the most basic and leading to more complex procedures and tests. In all cases of lung cancer diagnosis, a series of tests will be performed, rather than just one test. Usually, a team of physicians works together to determine a plan for a patient. The group may consist of a pulmonologist (lung specialist), a chest radiologist (X-ray specialist), and a thoracic surgeon.

Because there are so many different diagnostic tests for lung cancer, the team must choose very carefully. Its decision must be based on many factors: How is the patient's overall health? Is the tumor located centrally in the chest or peripherally (along the outer edges of the lung area)? How large does the tumor appear to be? Does it appear that the tumor has already spread to other parts of the body? Each patient must receive a unique plan for diagnosis based on the answers to these questions and many others.

IMAGING TESTS

After learning about the patient's family history and performing a medical examination, the medical team uses imaging tests to determine whether a mass of cells is present in or near the lungs. An

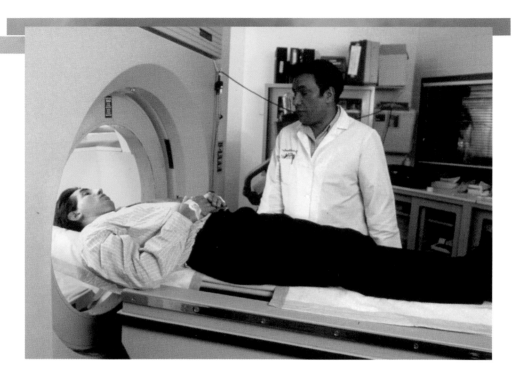

A patient undergoes a CT (computed tomography) scan in this image. According to a report on www.msnbc.com, CT scans are so effective in early detection of tumors, some physicians believe they should be performed annually on all patients with a history of lung cancer. But because the tests are expensive and not covered by many insurance carriers, this is not feasible for most people.

imaging test is one that uses X-rays, magnetic fields, sound waves, or radioactive substances to create a picture of the lungs. The first test to be performed is usually a chest X-ray. If no masses are visible in the lungs, the patient probably does not have lung cancer. In some instances, however, the X-ray may miss a tumor if it is less than 1 centimeter (0.39 inch) in diameter or if it is hidden behind a rib, collarbone, or the breastbone. If the radiologist observes anything suspicious, the patient will be recommended for a more advanced type of scan.

Researchers are currently developing new technology associated with chest X-rays. A digital chest X-ray uses a computerized detector rather than film. Sharper, clearer images are produced with this technique. Scientists are also experimenting with computers that "read" or analyze a chest X-ray. This technology is known as CAD, or computer-assisted diagnosis. The hope is that CAD may be able to detect more tumors than the human eye.

A CT (computed tomography) scan is really just a specialized X-ray machine. The CT scan is not only able to locate abnormal spots on the lungs like the chest X-ray, but it is also capable of providing much more exact information regarding the size, shape, and specific location of the tumor(s). Because the scanning machine rotates around the patient, the images it produces are three-dimensional. Layers of lung tissue are visible in very detailed cross sections. Most major hospitals today use a spiral, or helical, CT scan. Used since the 1990s, the spiral CT can scan a person's chest in less than thirty seconds.

From this point in their diagnosis, doctors have enough information about the tumor to proceed with more invasive procedures. The following diagnostic tests are used to determine whether a tumor is benign or malignant. If a tumor is determined to be malignant, one or more of the procedures will indicate the shape and composition of the cells, thereby confirming the type of lung cancer, SCLC or NSCLC.

SPUTUM ANALYSIS

Sputum is the material that is coughed up from the lungs. It may also be referred to as mucus, phlegm, or spit. One step in diagnosing lung cancer is a microscopic examination of the cells in the patient's sputum. The mucus generally is obtained through an instrument called a bronchoscope. The bronchoscope takes a sample of sputum directly from the lungs by sending a tube through the nose or mouth. Since this type of procedure is one of the least invasive, it is often the first option for

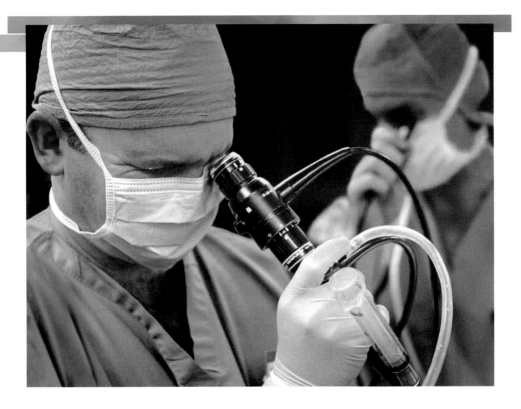

A pulmonologist performs a bronchoscopic biopsy. A flexible tube with a camera at its end is fed into a patient's mouth or nose and down to the lungs. Either forceps or a brush are then passed through the tube to collect tissue samples. This test can help physicians diagnose cancer and is less risky than surgery.

patients, especially those in weaker physical condition. Sputum analysis can diagnose, or detect, 30 percent of all lung cancers. If the results of the sputum analysis are not conclusive, a team of doctors will most likely follow up with other tests.

BIOPSY OF THE TUMOR

After the imaging tests are completed and the exact location and size of the tumor is determined, a sample of the cancerous cells will be

Once a physician has detected lung cancer in a patient, he or she may search for secondary tumors in order to make a fully informed diagnosis. A bone marrow aspiration, as shown in this photo, may be performed to see if cancer has spread to the patient's bones.

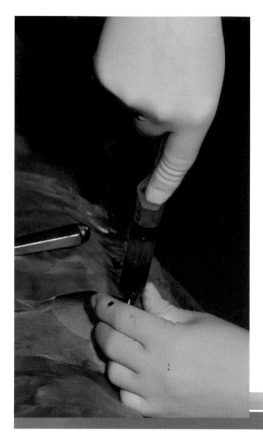

taken. The procedure for sampling a portion of a tumor is known as a biopsy. A pulmonary doctor obtains a sample of cells from the lungs, using one of the following methods. One method is bronchoscopy: just as a bronchoscope may be used to obtain mucus samples, it may also be used to collect cells in a tumor. Another method is called needle biopsy: a long needle is inserted through the chest wall to collect a sample of the tumor. A third method for obtaining a sample of the tumor is known as surgical biopsy: the chest wall is opened and the tumor is partially or entirely removed.

HAS THE CANCER SPREAD?

Typically, the last step in the diagnosis of lung cancer is to determine whether the cancer has spread, or metastasized, to other parts of the body. To locate additional secondary tumors, imaging scans such as the CT scan, MRI (magnetic resonance imaging), or bone scan may be performed, focusing on other parts of the body. Many other tests are available as well, each targeting a different part of the body. For example, blood tests may be done to determine if a person's liver and kidneys are properly functioning. A bone marrow biopsy may be done if there is reason to suspect the cancer has spread through the blood to the bones. When one or more secondary tumors are identified, doctors take on the task of assessing the patient's overall diagnosis.

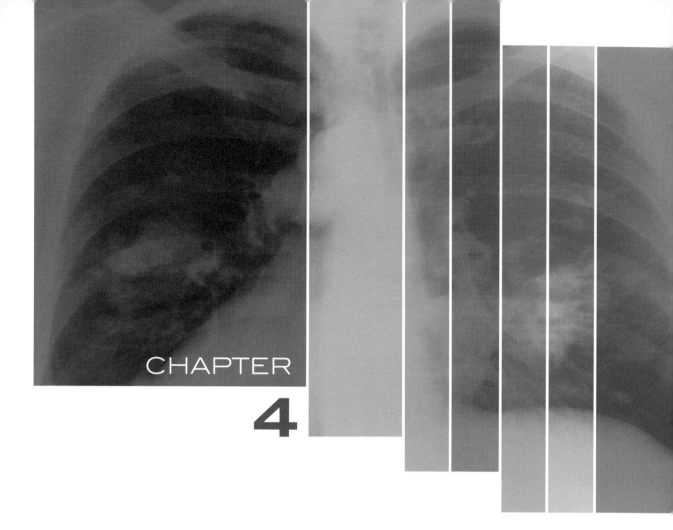

CHAPTER
4

TREATMENT OF
LUNG CANCER

Once a person is diagnosed with lung cancer, he or she must consult an oncologist, or cancer specialist, to plan treatment. The type of treatment a doctor recommends depends on a few factors: the patient's general health, the type of cancer, the size and location of the tumor in the lungs, and the extent to which the cancer has spread.

SURGERY

One option for some patients with lung cancer is surgical removal of a tumor. Surgery may be successful if the tumor is relatively small. There are three basic types of surgical procedures to remove tumors on the lungs. The first type of surgery is called wedge resection. In this operation, a small part of the lung is removed. Wedge resection works well if the tumor is centralized in a small area and if the cancer has not metastasized yet. Another method of surgery is known as a lobectomy. In this procedure, one entire lobe of the lung is removed. The final and most drastic form of surgery is a pneumonectomy. Here, the entire lung is removed. This procedure is only necessary if the cancer has spread throughout the whole lung.

RADIATION THERAPY

Radiation is a high-energy X-ray that is capable of killing cancer cells. Radiation therapy may be a patient's only form of treatment, or it may be combined with other methods. Sometimes, radiation is helpful after a person has surgery; small areas of cancer cells that were too small to remove surgically can be killed with radiation. The amount of radiation a patient receives varies, depending upon the size and location of the tumor. Radiation is often successful at relieving symptoms such as pain, bleeding, and blockage of the airways.

There are two different types of radiation therapy. External beam radiation therapy delivers radiation from a machine positioned outside the body. Internal radiation therapy, also known as brachytherapy, places a small pellet of radioactive materials near the cancer site inside the body. To do this, a small tube is placed in the airway, or trachea, near the tumor. The radioactive pellets are inserted into the tube and allowed to sit for several hours before being removed. This type of treatment is particularly helpful in shrinking tumors that are blocking a person's airways, making it difficult for him or her to breathe. Scientists believe that brachytherapy may also be successful if pellets are placed inside the chest cavity during lung surgery. Research in this area is currently under way.

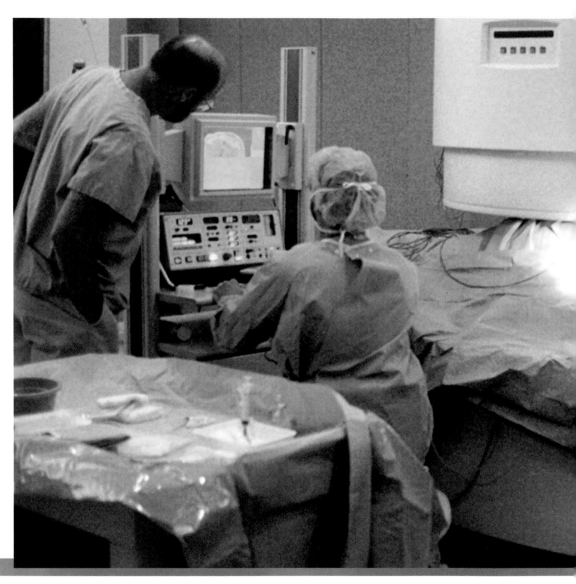

Above, external beam radiation is performed on a patient in Cleveland. The radiologist burns a cancerous tumor with radio waves while viewing his work on an MRI screen. Radiation therapy is most often used in conjunction with another treatment, such as surgery or chemotherapy, and it can also be used as pallia-tive therapy, to manage symptoms and relieve pain related to cancer.

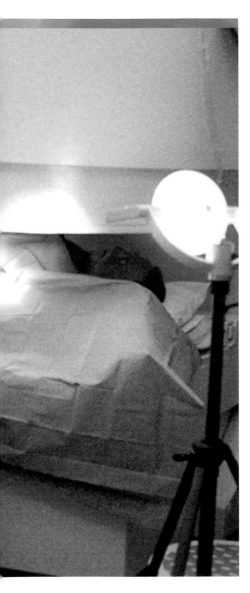

Researchers are constantly working on ways to improve radiation therapy. Radiosensitizers are substances that make the cancer cells more responsive to the effects of radiation. They may, for example, increase the oxygen level of the cancer cells. A tumor without enough oxygen is less likely to be killed by radiation. Experiments are also being conducted using radioprotectants. These are substances that protect the normal, healthy cells from radiation damage. Using radioprotectants may allow physicians to increase the total dose of radiation, thereby eliminating more of the cancer cells.

Both types of radiation therapy, whether delivered externally or internally, may result in side effects. The most severe symptoms include fatigue, upset stomach, diarrhea, and a skin rash. Many patients experience only mild side effects of radiation therapy such as a dry or sore throat and difficulty swallowing. A continual goal of lung cancer research is to experiment with the amount of radiation, combinations of the two types of radiation, and any other variables that may alleviate uncomfortable side effects.

CHEMOTHERAPY

Surgery and radiation therapy alone may be successful in the treatment of a patient whose lung cancer has been diagnosed early and has not spread to other parts of the body. Because the majority of lung cancers are not caught early enough, however, many patients require more aggressive treatments. After the cancer has metastasized beyond the lungs, the primary treatment is chemotherapy. The root word *chem-* means "chemical."

Various chemical drugs have been formulated to kill cancer cells. During chemotherapy, a patient receives a combination of these drugs. The drugs may enter the bloodstream either through injection or a pill. Using the blood vessels as their pathway, the drugs travel to all parts of the body, killing the cancer cells that have spread. In addition to killing cancer cells, however, these powerful drugs may also kill or damage healthy cells. The specific type of drugs and the amount, or dosage, are planned individually for each patient. As with the other treatments, the physician must consider many factors such as the type of lung cancer, the extent it has spread, and the age and health of the patient before prescribing chemotherapy.

Chemotherapy may be used in addition to surgery or radiation treatments for lung cancer. Chemotherapy is often recommended as the primary treatment in all stages of small cell lung cancer. Unfortunately, because chemotherapy drugs are so strong, they often result in severe side effects for the patient. A patient may experience one or more of the following symptoms: nausea or vomiting, hair loss, diarrhea, lack of energy, loss of appetite, and mouth sores. Among the healthy cells that may be damaged by chemotherapy are the blood-producing cells of the bone marrow. Without adequate numbers of blood cells, a patient may be more susceptible to infections, bleeding and bruising, fatigue, and shortness of breath.

Scientists are actively researching many new chemotherapy drugs and new techniques for delivering them. One area of research involves testing a drug on a small sample of a patient's cancer cells to determine its effectiveness. The patient would then avoid the side effects of a drug that wasn't working. Research is also being done to determine the effectiveness of inhaling chemotherapy drugs directly into the airways. Targeted therapy is a new method for designing drugs to act specifically on cancer cells, rather than acting on *any* cells that are dividing quickly. Yet another new area of research involves substances that are able to cut off the blood supply to a tumor. Without blood, cancer cells cannot continue to grow and multiply.

CLINICAL TRIALS

Another option for lung cancer patients is known as a clinical trial. The term "trial" indicates that this type of treatment is experimental and completely optional for the patient. Typically, a patient participating in a clinical trial will be testing a new type of drug. One drug may be incorporated into a patient's chemotherapy. Another drug may help to boost the patient's immune system. For example, the experimental drug may be able to recognize abnormal substances in cancer cells. Yet another type of clinical trial may involve genetics, altering a patient's DNA due to mutations that have caused his or her cells to become cancerous. Any new medicine, technique, or therapy of any sort must go through a series of clinical trials in order to be proven effective.

Clinical trials are divided into three distinct phases, each designed to serve a different purpose. In the case of a new drug, all three phases must be successfully completed before the U.S. Food and Drug Administration (FDA) will approve it and make it available for the public. Each phase of a clinical trial takes place separately, one at a time. For instance, phase II may not begin until the results of phase I are satisfactory. The trial may not progress to phase III until the results of phase II are complete and acceptable. In some cases, a phase IV clinical trial is conducted after the FDA approves the drug. The number of participants increases with each phase. Typically, only 10 to 20 people are enrolled in a phase I trial, 20 to 200 people in a phase II trial, and 200 to 1,000

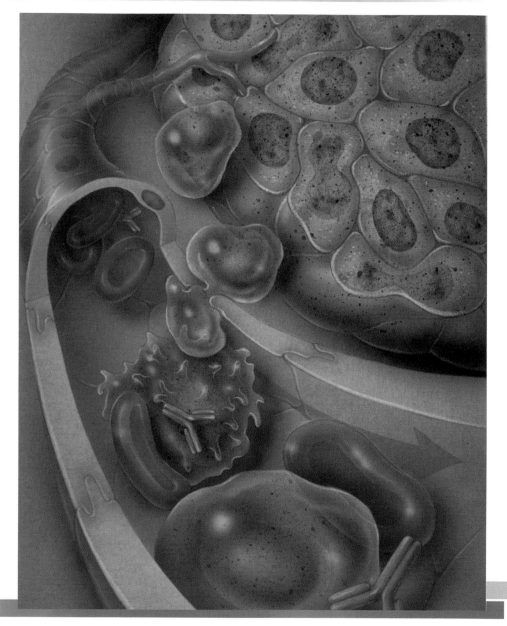

This schematic represents the metastatic process. The spread and growth of cancerous tumors is important for physicians to discover and researchers to study, because a large portion of cancer fatalities are linked to secondary, rather than primary, tumors. Developing a method of cutting the blood supply to a tumor may be a solution.

people in a phase III clinical trial. The greater the number of participants, the more conclusive the results will be.

In phase I of a clinical trial, researchers test the basic safety of a new drug. The most effective method for administering the drug and the proper dosage will be determined in this part of the clinical trial. Drugs may be given orally (by mouth), injected into the bloodstream, injected into the muscle, or in new experimental cases, inhaled. Scientists must determine which method is safest and most effective for the particular drug being tested. The dosage of a drug includes how often the drug should be taken and how much of the drug should be taken. The goal is to determine the most effective dose that is still safe for the patient. The final purpose of a phase I clinical trial is to learn about any harmful side effects caused by the new drug.

As soon as phase I is successfully completed, the clinical trial moves on to phase II. One purpose of a phase II clinical trial is simply to continue the work begun in phase I—evaluating the safety of the drug. Researchers will also study how the body metabolizes the drug. How well is the drug absorbed into the cells? How well does the drug pass safely through the body? In addition to answering these questions, scientists will also begin to collect data about the effectiveness of the drug: does the drug do what it is supposed to do? If the results of a phase II clinical trial confirm the safety of the drug and if the drug appears to be effective, the process moves forward to a phase III trial.

Phase III is designed to compare the new treatment being tested in the clinical trial with a standard treatment already available on the market. There are at least two types of treatment, called arms, involved in a phase III trial. People placed in the experimental treatment arm receive the new drug. People placed in the control arm receive the best treatment available to the public. Participants are selected for one arm or the other at random. They cannot choose which group they are placed in, nor will they be told which treatment they are receiving. This is known as a blinded trial. Phase III clinical trials enroll the largest number of people, are randomized, and are blinded to increase the validity of the results. The more valid the results are, the more likely the FDA is to approve the drug for public use.

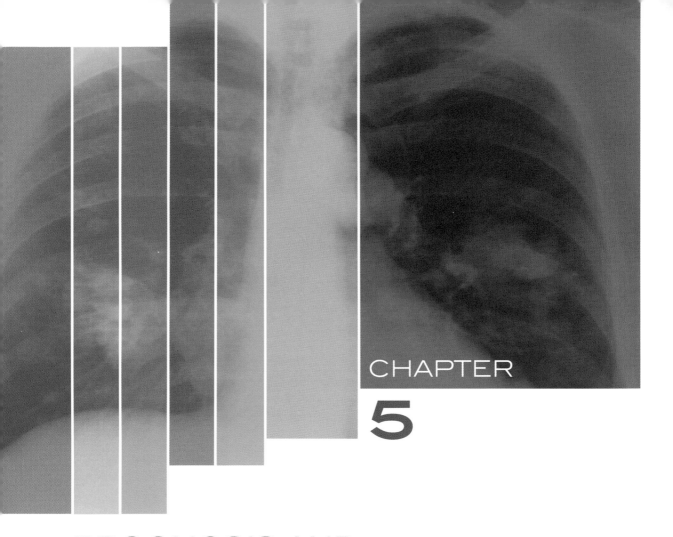

CHAPTER

5

PROGNOSIS AND PREVENTION

After a lung cancer patient has undergone treatment, an oncologist will determine a prognosis, or prediction of his or her future health. Oncologists often indicate a patient's prognosis by the number of years they believe the patient will live after diagnosis. A five-year survival rate, for example, refers to the percentage of patients who will live at least five years after they are diagnosed with lung cancer. A one-year survival rate would most likely categorize patients in the most advanced stages of lung cancer.

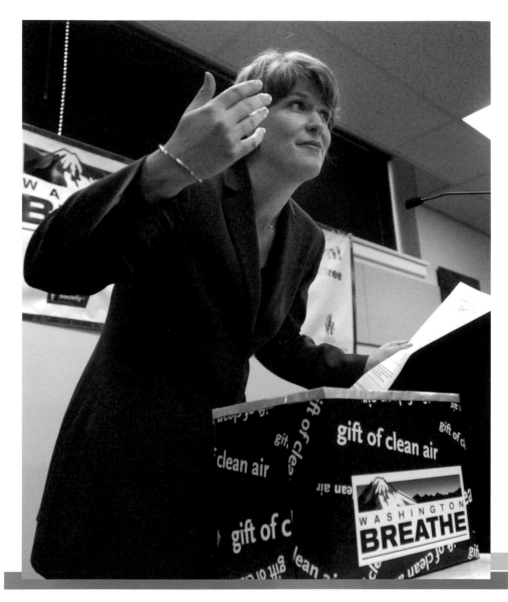

Now that specific causes of lung cancer have been pinpointed, much is being done to prevent the disease. Here, the chief executive officer of the American Lung Association holds a press conference to urge state legislatures to ban smoking in public places. Employees of bars, restaurants, and other venues where smoking is allowed are at greater risk for developing lung cancer.

STATISTICS

Various organizations periodically conduct national surveys in order to collect data about lung cancer patients. The American Cancer Society most recently compiled lung cancer data nationally in 1998. At that time, the five-year survival rate for all types and all stages of lung cancer combined was 15 percent. This means that only 15 percent of patients diagnosed with lung cancer were expected to live five years or more. The average one-year survival rate, determined in the same study, was 42 percent. Both of these statistics were found to be very consistent in recent years. The one-year survival rate, in fact, had not changed for ten years, since 1988. Ten years prior, however, in 1978, the one-year survival rate was approximately 30 percent. This improvement in the survival rate was most likely due to technological and medical advances, especially in the field of surgery.

The American Cancer Society study also provided data regarding the survival rate of patients whose lung cancer was detected before spreading to other parts of the body. Recall that only about 15 percent of all the types of lung cancers combined are detected this early. In those cases, the patient's five-year survival rate jumps to 48 percent. This means that almost half of lung cancer patients who are diagnosed in the early stages will live at least five more years.

Perhaps the most frightening statistic regarding lung cancer is the dramatic increase in the number of deaths over the years. According to the American Lung Association (ALA), the number of deaths caused by lung cancer in 1950 was 18,000; in 1984, the number rose to 115,000; and by 1994, lung cancer deaths reached 142,000. The ALA predicted that the number for 2004 would be 160,000. Obviously, medical, genetic, and technological advances cannot keep up with the risk factors that still exist.

METHODS OF PREVENTION

Research is currently being conducted at medical centers worldwide in order to find ways to fight lung cancer. Many believe that the most lives will be saved if new methods of prevention are available. Because cigarette smoking is the greatest risk factor by far (85 percent of all lung cancers are the result of carcinogens in tobacco) for developing lung cancer, the bulk of this research focuses on ways to either help people quit smoking or to convince people not to start smoking in the first place.

QUIT SMOKING

The growing number of lung cancer–related deaths directly corresponds with the rise in cigarette smoking over the years. The leading risk factor for lung cancer, cigarette smoking, is also the most preventable. Just stop smoking! Because cigarettes are highly addictive, however, this is much easier to say than to do. Nicotine is the addictive substance found in tobacco. The surgeon general has compared nicotine addiction to the addiction experienced with heroin and cocaine. Researchers continue to search for ways to help people put an end to their strong nicotine addictions.

One promising method used to help smokers quit is called nicotine replacement therapy (NRT). Doses of nicotine are placed in patches worn on the skin, in chewing gum, in the mist of an inhaler, or in nasal spray. These various methods temporarily replace the nicotine in cigarettes with nicotine from another source. NRT has proven to ease the physical withdrawal symptoms that people experience when they stop smoking. If the symptoms that accompanied quitting smoking weren't so severe, more people would be successful. Trouble sleeping, mood changes, headaches, restlessness, and irritability are just a few of the symptoms associated with nicotine withdrawal. The theory behind NRT is that if these difficult symptoms are alleviated, the

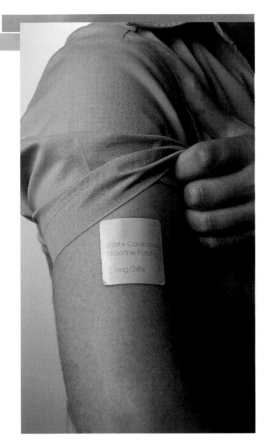

Smoking is difficult to quit. Because nicotine is addictive, quitting cold turkey can seem impossible. That's why many physicians prescribe nicotine gums, candies, and patches, like the one shown here. The patch works by releasing measured amounts of nicotine into the wearer's bloodstream so that he or she doesn't experience drastic withdrawal. The idea is to taper nicotine doses and to eventually eliminate the wearer's need for nicotine altogether. Nicotine patches have proven to be extremely successful.

smoker will have an easier time giving up cigarettes.

Nicotine replacement therapy has proven to work well. According to a study reported in the 2001 issue of *American Family Physician*, smokers who used NRT were 2.27 times more likely to quit than those who didn't try the therapy. Additionally, the rate of success (the proportion of smokers who are able to quit) is doubled within the first six to twelve months when using NRT. Most physicians recommend counseling or classes in addition to NRT. No medication is without risk, however. NRT, especially if an improper dose is taken, may cause side effects such as nausea, abdominal pain, headache, dizziness, difficulty breathing, heart palpitations, and in severe cases, depression. With the exception of nicotine gum and certain types of patches, most NRT is available only by prescription. Consulting a doctor is crucial before beginning any therapy to quit smoking.

The good news is that in many cases, the negative effects of smoking can reverse themselves over time. Ten years after a person stops smoking, his or her risk for developing lung cancer drops by one-third. Any time a smoker quits before cancer develops, there is good news; new, healthy lung cells form and gradually take the place of all the damaged cells.

TEST HOME FOR RADON

Radon, the invisible, odorless gas found in soil, rock, and groundwater, is responsible for 12 percent of all lung cancers. This statistic alone should motivate people to have their homes tested for radon. In addition to being inexpensive, do-it-yourself radon testing kits are quick and easy to use. They can be purchased by mail, through the Internet, or in certain hardware stores. If a test indicates radon levels above 4 picocuries per liter (4 pCi/L), steps should be taken to reduce radon levels in the home. The solution may be as simple as sealing cracks in floors and walls. In other homes, it may be necessary to set up a soil suction system. (A soil suction system is a simple system using pipes and fans to reduce the radon in a building.) In order to prevent high radon levels in a new home, special construction techniques may be effective. These radon-resistant methods are easy and inexpensive and should help to reduce the indoor radon level of the new building.

QUESTION WORKPLACE ENVIRONMENT

All workplaces should be up-to-date with federal regulations regarding certain carcinogens, such as asbestos. Laws have been put in place to protect workers from most cancer-causing substances, but some of these substances are still present. For example, people who work with machines or vehicles that require diesel fuel inhale exhaust along with air. Workers in conditions like this should try to find ways to limit or completely avoid their exposure to any carcinogens in the air. Additional advice would be

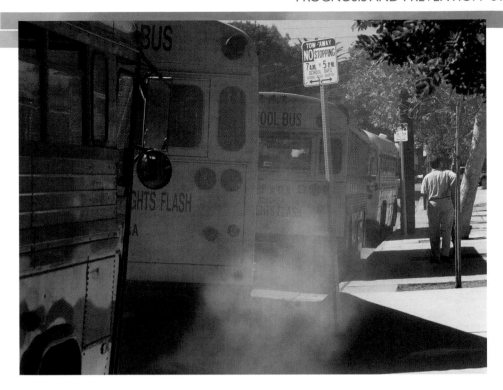

Twenty-four million American children spend an average of 1.5 hours every school day on a bus. Since about 90 percent of U.S. school buses run on diesel fuel, bus drivers and schoolchildren are getting too much exposure to a potentially deadly carcinogen. Cleaner buses will be available in 2007, and new technology has been developed to reduce carcinogenic emissions in the older buses that will still be in use.

to stay aware of current research and environmental laws concerning any of the carcinogens that may be in the workplace.

SCREENING

Screening is the use of tests or examinations to detect a disease in people who do not have any symptoms of the disease. However, not just anyone is eligible for screening. In the case of lung cancer, people who are exposed to any of the risk factors may be screened for the disease. Currently, screening procedures are experimental. Researchers are

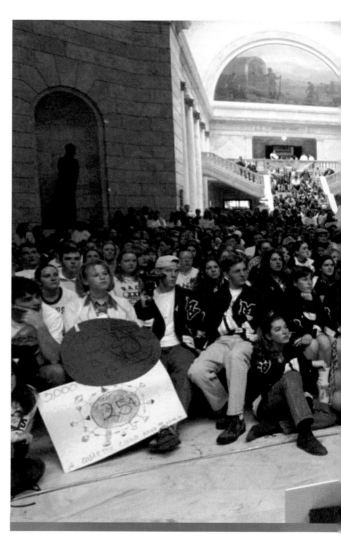

One of the greatest battles in the war on lung cancer is educating the public, specifically children, about smoking. As shown in this photo, most elementary and secondary schools host rallies and assemblies at least once a year to teach students about the potentially fatal consequences of smoking. Often, these are held in November on the day of the Great American Smokeout, when smokers are encouraged to put their habit on hold.

designing clinical trials to screen certain people at risk for lung cancer. They will then analyze the data to determine whether screening will catch the disease in earlier stages, resulting in a higher survival rate. Lung cancer screening will not become a routine practice until the research proves that it will save lives.

Lung cancer, the leading cancer killer worldwide, is a hot topic of current research. However, despite research in areas such as early diagnosis and prevention, the number of lung cancer deaths continues to grow dramatically every year. Why is this killer spreading so rapidly when it is by far the most preventable type of cancer? Eighty-five percent of all lung cancer deaths can be directly linked to the carcinogens in cigarette smoke. What type of

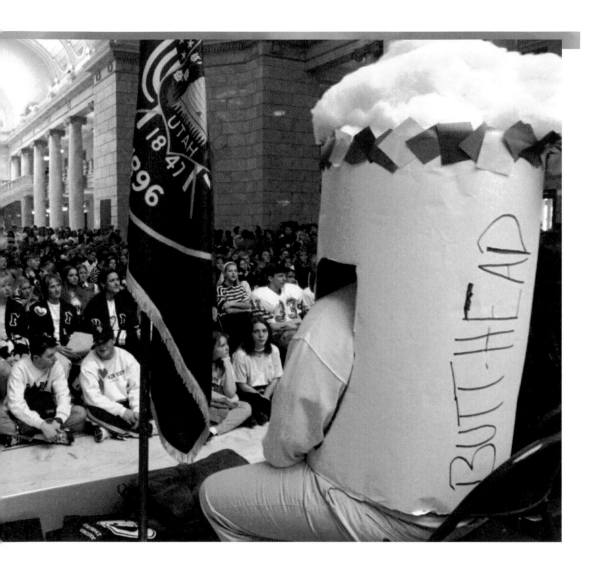

research will actually stop people from falling prey to this leading risk factor? Scientists and educators must unite forces in order to tackle these questions. Convincing people of all ages around the globe not to start smoking is the first key to lowering the lung cancer death toll. The second, perhaps more challenging goal of current research is to help smokers quit.

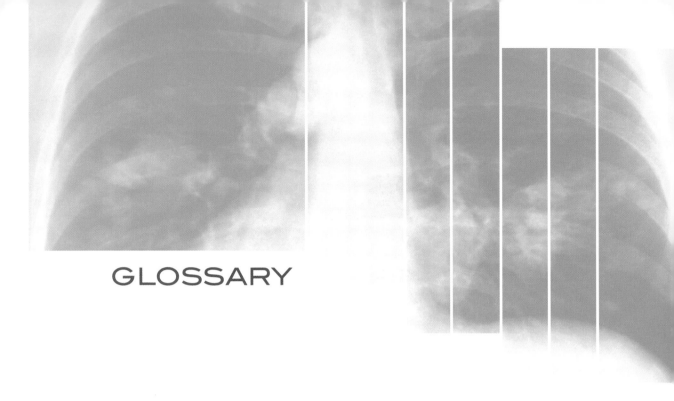

GLOSSARY

alveoli Tiny air sacs responsible for respiration in the lungs. Here, oxygen is absorbed into the bloodstream.

benign Refers to a tumor that is noncancerous and, therefore, not life threatening.

biopsy The process of sampling a portion of a tumor.

blinded trial A clinical trial in which the participants do not know if they are receiving the standard treatment or the experimental treatment.

brachytherapy The process of placing a small pellet of radioactive material near the cancer site; internal radiation.

bronchi Tubes that bring air from the end of the trachea (windpipe) to smaller tubes called bronchioles.

bronchioles Many tiny tubes that bring air from the bronchi to alveoli (air sacs).

carcinogen Any cancer-causing agent.

carcinoma Any cancerous tumor.

chemotherapy A treatment for cancer involving a combination of drugs.

cross section An image showing a layer, or slice, through a three-dimensional object.

esophagus The tube that brings food from the mouth to the stomach.

gland Any organ or group of cells that produces and secretes some substance, such as sweat, urine, or a hormone.

lymphatic system The group of structures responsible for filtering out foreign particles such as viruses, bacteria, and cancer cells.

malignant Refers to a cancerous tumor that has the potential of spreading.

mesothelioma The type of lung cancer caused by exposure to asbestos.

metastasis The process by which cancer cells spread to other parts of the body.

mitosis The process by which one body cell divides, creating two new cells identical to the first.

mucin A thick liquid secreted by adenocarcinoma cells.

mutation A change in the genetic material (DNA) of a cell.

oncologist A physician specializing in cancer.

pleura The protective, moist lining surrounding the lungs.

prognosis The prediction of future health status.

trachea The windpipe; the tube that brings air from the mouth to the lungs.

tumor A group of cells resulting from abnormal cell division.

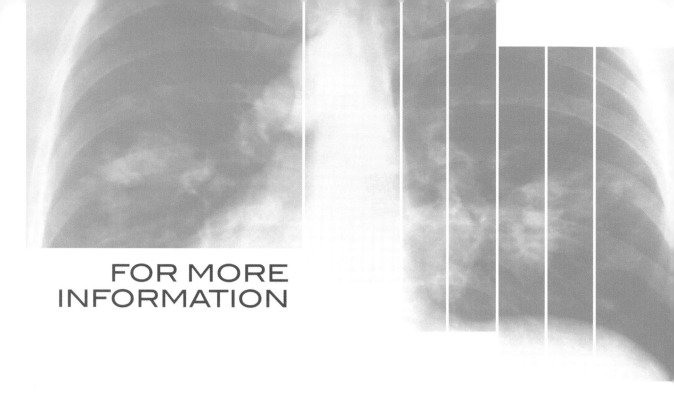

FOR MORE INFORMATION

Alliance for Lung Cancer Advocacy, Support, and Education (ALCASE)
1155 21st Street NW, Suite 350
Washington, DC 20036
(800) 298-2436 (United States only)
Web site: http://www.alcase.org

American Cancer Society
1599 Clifton Road NE
Atlanta, GA 30329
(800) 227-2345
Web site: http://www.cancer.org

American Lung Association
1740 Broadway
New York, NY 10019-4374
(800) 586-4872 or (212) 315-8700
Web site: http://www.lungusa.org

National Cancer Institute (National Institutes of Health)
9000 Rockville Pike
Bethesda, MD 20892
(800) 4-CANCER (422-6237)
Web site: http://www.nci.nih.gov or www.cancer.gov

IN CANADA
Canadian Cancer Society
National Office
10 Alcorn Avenue, Suite 200
Toronto, ON
M4V 3B1
(416) 961-7223
Web site: http://www.cancer.ca/ccs

Canadian Lung Association
3 Raymond Street, Suite 300
Ottawa, ON
K1R 1A3
(613) 569-6411
Web site: http://www.lung.ca

WEB SITES
Due to the changing nature of Internet links, the Rosen Publishing
Group, Inc., has developed an online list of Web sites related to the
subject of this book. This site is updated regularly. Please use this link
to access the list:

http://www.rosenlinks.com/cms/luca

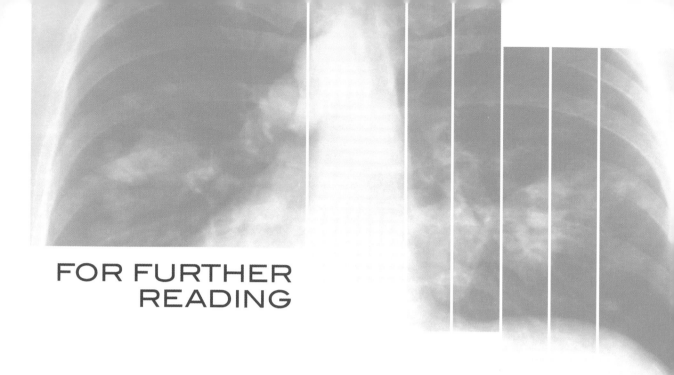

FOR FURTHER READING

Brill, Marlene Targ. *Lung Cancer.* Health Alert Series. New York, NY: Benchmark Books, 2005.

Caldwell, Wilma R., et al. *Cancer Information for Teens: Health Tips About Cancer Awareness, Prevention, Diagnosis and Treatment.* Teen Health Series. Detroit, MI: Omnigraphics, 2004.

Cox, Barbara G., David T. Carr, and Robert E. Lee. *Living with Lung Cancer: A Guide for Patients and Their Families.* Gainsville, FL: Triad Publishing Company, 1998.

Henschke, Claudia I., Peggy McCarthy, and Sarah Wernick. *Lung Cancer: Myths, Facts, Choices—and Hope.* New York, NY: W. W. Norton & Company, 2003.

Johnston, Lorraine. *Lung Cancer: Making Sense of Diagnosis, Treatment and Options.* Cambridge, MA: O'Reilly Publishing Company, 2001.

Kittredge, Mary. *The Respiratory System.* Encyclopedia of Health, the Human Body. Langhorne, PA: Chelsea House Publishers, 2000.

Parles, Karen, and Joan H. Schiller. *100 Questions & Answers About Lung Cancer.* Boston, MA: Jones & Bartlett Publishing, 2002.

St. John, Tina. *With Every Breath: A Lung Cancer Guidebook.* Vancouver, WA: Alliance for Lung Cancer Advocacy, Support, and Education, 2003.

Walter, Scott. *Lung Cancer: A Guide to Diagnosis and Treatment.* Omaha, NE: Addicus Books, 2001.

Ward, Jeremy P. T., et al. *The Respiratory System at a Glance.* Malden, MA: Blackwell Publishers, 2002.

Yount, Lisa. *Cancer.* Lucent Overview Series. San Diego, CA: Greenhaven Press, 1999.

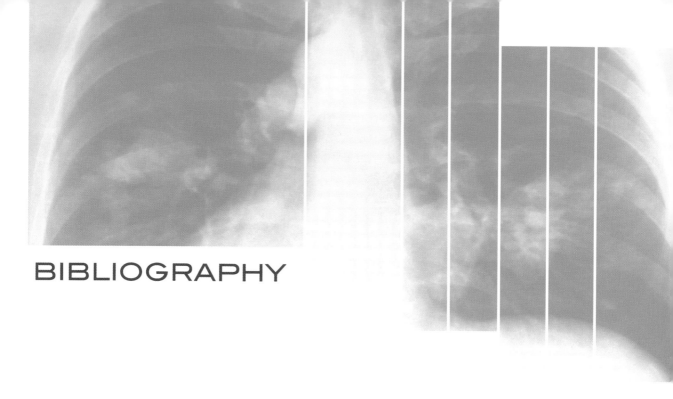

BIBLIOGRAPHY

American Cancer Society. "Cancer Reference Information." 2003. Retrieved April 2, 2004 (http://www.cancer.org).

American Cancer Society. "Early Detection Trial for Current and Former Smokers." 2004. Retrieved August 5, 2004 (http://www.cancer.org).

American Cancer Society. "Lung Cancer." 2004. Retrieved April 2, 2004 (http://www.cancer.org).

American Lung Association. "Facts About Lung Cancer." 2003. Retrieved March 25, 2004 (http://www.lungusa.org).

Cherath, Lata. "Lung Cancer," in *Gale Encyclopedia of Medicine*. Farmington Hills, MI: Gale Group, 1999.

Microsoft Encarta. "Lung Cancer." 2004. Retrieved March 25, 2004 (http://encarta.msn.com).

Mirken, Bruce. "Nicotine Replacement Therapy." 2001. Retrieved August 5, 2004 (http://www.ahealthyme.com).

National Human Genome Research Institute and National Institutes of Health. "Location of Potential Familial Lung Cancer

Gene Discovered." 2004. Retrieved August 5, 2004 (http://www.nhgri.nih.gov).

St. John, Tina. *With Every Breath: A Lung Cancer Guidebook.* Vancouver, WA: Alliance for Lung Cancer Advocacy, Support, and Education, 2003.

United States Environmental Protection Agency. "A Citizen's Guide to Radon." 4th ed. 2002. Retrieved August 5, 2004 (http://www.epa.gov/iaq/radon/pubs/citiguide.html).

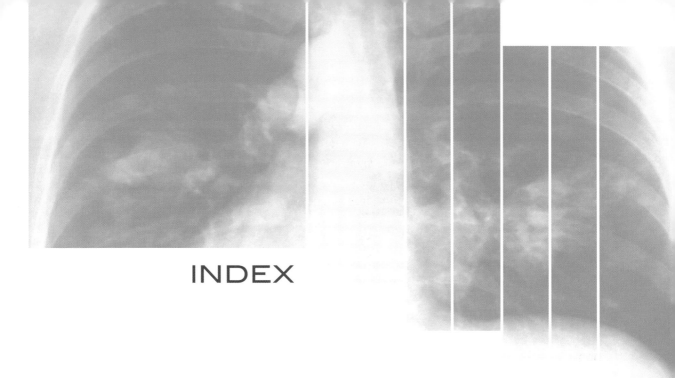

INDEX

ABOUT THE AUTHOR
Julie Walker is a seventh-grade life science teacher in Sudbury, Massachusetts. She has a B.A. in biology and an M.A. in education.

PHOTO CREDITS
Cover, pp. 8, 31, 34 © Custom Medical Stock Photo, Inc.; cover corner photo © PunchStock; back cover and throughout © National Cancer Institute; p. 5 © Ernst Tobisch/Unep/Peter Arnold, Inc.; p. 10 © Ed Reschke/Peter Arnold, Inc.; p. 12 © St. Bartholomew's Hospital/Photo Researchers, Inc.; p. 13 © Russell Kightley Media; p. 16 © Sheri Blaney/Index Stock Imagery; pp. 18–19 © Sonda Dawes/The Image Works; p. 21 © Ted Spiegel/ Corbis; p. 22 © Van Miller/Index Stock Imagery; p. 23 © David Duprey/AP/Wide World Photos; p. 25 © Stief & Schnare/SuperStock; p. 29 © Dave L. Ryan/Index Stock Imagery; p. 33 © Lester Lefkowitz/ Corbis; pp. 38–39 © Elizabeth Malby, The Plain Dealer/AP/ Wide World Photos; p. 42 © Kevin A. Somerville/ Phototake; p. 46 © Elaine Thompson/AP/Wide World Photos; p. 49 © Photolibrary/Index Stock Imagery; p. 51 © Mark J.Terrill/AP/Wide World Photo; pp. 52–53 © Douglas C. Pizac/AP/Wide World Photos.

Designer: Evelyn Horovicz; Editor: Christine Poolos